Weight Watchers Instant Pot Smart Points Cookbook:

The Complete Weight Watchers Instant Pot Cookbook - with 60 Healthy & Delicious Instant Pot Cooker Recipes

By Mirna Merritt

© Copyright 2016 by Mirna Merritt - All rights reserved.

This document is geared towards providing exact and reliable information in regards to the topic and issue covered. The publication is sold with the idea that the publisher is not required to render accounting, officially permitted, or otherwise, qualified services. If advice is necessary, legal or professional, a practiced individual in the profession should be ordered.

Under no circumstance will any legal responsibility or blame be held against the publisher for any reparation, damages, or monetary loss due to the information herein, either directly or indirectly.

Legal Notice:

The book is copyright protected. This is only for personal use. You cannot amend, distribute, sell, use, quote or paraphrase any part or the content within this book without the consent of the author.

Disclaimer Notice:

Please note the information contained within this document is for educational and entertainment purposes only. Every attempt has been made to provide accurate, up to date and reliable complete information. No warranties of any kind are expressed or implied. Readers acknowledge that the author is not engaging in the rendering of legal, financial, medical or professional advice. The content of this book has been derived from various sources. Please consult a licensed professional before attempting any techniques outlined in this book.

By reading this document, the reader agrees that under no circumstances are is the author responsible for any loses, direct or indirect, which are incurred as a result the use of information contained within this document, including, but not limited to, —errors, omissions, or inaccuracies.

Table of Contents

Introduction to Weight Watchers Diet..................................8
What Are Smartpoints?...9
Pros and Cons of Smartpoints..10
    Advantages..10
    Disadvantages...11
10 Mistakes When Using Instant Pot Cooker....................12
Soup and Stew Recipes...15
    Instant Pot Vegetable Soup..15
    Low Fat Taco Soup..17
    Five Can Soup..19
    Instant Pot Tomato Spinach Soup.................................20
    French Onion Soup..22
    Cheeseburger Stew...24
    Instant Pot Broccoli Cheese Soup.................................26
    Cheesy Potato Soup with Bacon...................................27
    Cauliflower and Broccoli Soup......................................29
    Baked Potato Soup..31
    Broccoli Potato Cheese Chowder..................................33
    Egg Drop Soup with Chicken.......................................35

Chicken Recipes... 36
- Parmesan Chicken with Mushroom and Wine Sauce.... 36
- Instant Pot Sweet and Sour Chicken.............................. 38
- Steamed Jalapeno Chicken.. 40
- Steamed Coconut Chicken with Pina Colada Dip.......... 41
- Instant Pot Roast Chicken.. 43
- Steamed Chicken Pot Pie... 45
- Chicken Steak.. 47
- Steamed Lemon Chicken Breast.................................... 48
- Sesame Chicken.. 49
- Instant Pot Teriyaki Chicken.. 51
- Instant Pot Curried Lemon Coconut Chicken................ 52
- One Pot Chicken Cacciatore.. 53

Beef Recipes.. 55
- Instant Pot Caribbean Pineapple Filet Mignon.............. 55
- Ground Beef and Cabbage Casserole............................ 57
- Instant Pot Meatloaf... 59
- Instant Pot Lasagna.. 61
- Beef Taco Rice.. 63
- Herb-Crusted Beef.. 65
- Instant Pot Mexican Beef.. 66
- Instant Pot Salisbury Steak... 68
- Beef Stroganoff... 70

Barbacoa Beef 72

Tomato Beef Macaroni Soup 74

Tropical Beef with Peppers and Pineapple 76

Pork Recipes 78

Steamed Pork Tenderloin with Herbs 78

Southwestern Pork Chops 80

BBQ Pork Tenderloin with Mop Sauce 81

Pork Chop Stew 83

Instant Pot Balsamic Pork Roast 85

Pork Carnitas 87

Teriyaki Pork Tenderloin 89

Pork with Salsa 91

Pork Tenderloin Green Chili 93

Apple Barbecue Ribs 95

Honey Balsamic Pork Roast 96

Apple Bacon BBQ Pulled Pork 97

Dessert Recipes 99

Mini Flourless Peanut Butter Chocolate Cakes 99

Instant Pot Berry Cobbler 101

Scalloped Peaches 103

Custard Cream Cheesecake 104

Instant Pot Applesauce 106

Thai Coconut Rice 108

Toffee Pudding...110

Apple Crisps..112

Chocolate Berry Cheesecake..114

Molten Chocolate Mini Lava Cake..................................117

Pumpkin Banana Chocolate Chip Bundt Cake..............119

Apple Bread with Salted Caramel Icing.........................121

Introduction to Weight Watchers Diet

There are different types of diet regimens that promise a lot of health benefits. One of the diet regimens that you can follow to lose weight is the Weight Watchers diet. The Weight Watchers diet is a lifestyle-change program as it imparts dieters to eat healthier and engage in physical activities in order to lose weight.

The Weight Watchers is a membership diet program that offers you different services such as exercise programs, recipes, weekly meeting schedule, and one-on-one consultations. Unlike other types of diet regimens, Weight Watchers does not restrict dieters from eating certain foods thereby making this diet program great for people with different types of food preference.

The Weight Watchers is designed to provide dieters with all the help that they need in order to adapt to a healthier lifestyle. Part of the Weight Watchers diet program is learning about how to shop and cook healthy foods by yourself.

Although the program also includes delivery of packaged foods, members are not strictly required to take this option. Another important facet of the Weight Watchers is that members can attend in-person meeting to learn more tips and tricks about dieting and weight loss. Moreover, they can also keep track of their progress with the app that is included with the program.

The Weight Watchers is one of the most popular weight loss regimens available today. In fact, there have been several studies that have shown that it can help lose and maintain weight properly. But more than losing weight, there are a lot of benefits of Weight Watchers. In fact, this diet program can benefit people who suffer from high cholesterol, high blood pressure, heart diseases, and diabetes.

What Are Smartpoints?

What makes Weight Watchers unique is its smartpoints counting system. This counting system is based on the amount of saturated fat, calories, proteins, and sugar found in ingredients used in making food. The value looks at the calorie count first and it increases with the presence of fat and sugar. However, the value of the smartpoints lowers with the presence of proteins. Below are things to remember regarding the smartpoints.

- Every food is assigned its own smartpoints value.

- Fruits and most vegetables are assigned zero points.
- Different people get different smartpoints budget assigned during the first consultation with weight watchers.

The thing is that when you join Weight Watchers, you will be assigned your very own smartpoint budget based on your gender, height, weight, and age. The smartpoint budget makes up your daily and weekly allowances so that you can easily plan your meals, make healthy choices, and splurge only if your smartpoints budget allows it.

Pros and Cons of Smartpoints

While the Weight Watchers smartpoints is a great way to keep track of the types of foods that you eat, there are benefits and downsides Below are the advantages and disadvantages to this calorie counting system.

Advantages

- Smartpoints is all about encouraging people to create healthier food choices instead of focusing on calorie counting. It encourages dieters to eat food with more protein and less refined sugar and carbohydrates.

- Unlike the previous counting system, the smartpoints does not eat your fitpoints. Fitpoints refer to the points that you get when you add physical activities and exercises. Under the old counting system, your points diminish as your physical activities also increase. Unfortunately, this results to people making unhealthy choices with the food they are going to spend on their extra points. With smartpoints, they are separated so you can continue making healthy food choices.

Disadvantages

- While the benefit of smartpoints is to genuinely transform people into adapting into healthy lifestyle. Unfortunately, it is difficult for most people to make such adjustment. This is especially true if they have gotten used to the old counting system – the PointsPlus.

- Smartpoints impose stricter penalties when eating food high in sugar and saturated fats. In fact, smartpoints value foods with higher points compared to the older system.

- Since smartpoints is stricter than the older system, it can cause some dieters to lose their willpower to follow it.

10 Mistakes When Using Instant Pot Cooker

There are many Weight Watchers recipes that you can make with an Instant Pot. As a third generation of digital pressure cookers, Instant Pot allows you to cook healthier food at a faster time. If you are planning on using your Instant Pot to prepare Weight Watcher friendly recipes, then there are certain things you need to remember to create healthy and delicious meals all the time. Below are the 10 common mistakes when using your Instant Pot cooker and how to avoid them.

1. **Forgetting to place the inner pot inside the Instant Pot before pouring the ingredients:** The inner pot is a very important component of the Instant Pot. Dumping the ingredients without the inner pot can damage the electronic components of the pot.

2. **Putting too much ingredients:** Many users stretch the capabilities of their Instant Pot by putting too much ingredients (particularly liquid) up to Max Line. This will risk clogging the venting knob that allows the excess pressure from escaping the pot. If

you overfill the pot, do natural release instead of a quick release because this will further the clogging.

3. **Using quick release when cooking foamy food:** Foamy foods like beans and grains can clog the venting knob and also produce splatter of hot liquid. Make sure that you do natural release when you are cooking them.

4. **Pressing the timer button to set the cooking time:** Remember that the timer button is used for delayed cooking. So, do not press on this button unless you want to cook your food on a later time. If you did press this button, press on the Keep Warm/Cancel button to stop the timer.

5. **Forgetting to turn the venting knob to the sealing position:** The venting knob should be closed to create a pressured environment. If you don't turn it to the sealing position, you are as good as cooking from an ordinary pot.

6. **Putting the Instant Pot on top of the stove and turning the dial on:** The Instant Pot already comes with its own heating element so you don't need to put it on top of a stove. If you do, you are just burning the bottom.

7. **Cooking with not enough liquid:** The Instant Pot uses steam to increase the pressure. Not cooking with enough liquid prevents pressure from building up inside the pot. It is recommended to use at least w cup of liquid when cooking food. If you are adding thickeners like starches, make sure that you put them after the pressure cooking cycle.

8. **Not putting the sealing ring back in the lid:** The sealing ring prevents the steam from escaping the pot thus this prevents the pot from building the pressure it needs to cook faster. Make it a habit to always check if the sealing ring is placed in the lid.

9. **Using the rice button for cooking all types of rice:** While the rice button is designed to cook rice, not all rice can be cooked with this preset button. When cooking different types of rice, use the manual button instead.

10. **Using hot liquid even if the recipe calls for cold liquid:** What is the difference if you use hot liquid when the recipe calls for cold? What happens is that it affects the cooking time of your food. When you use hot liquid, the cooking time will become shorter as the inner pot takes less time to come into the right pressure.

Soup and Stew Recipes

Instant Pot Vegetable Soup

Yields: 1
Cooking time: 10 minutes
Preparation time: 5 minutes

Nutritional Information per Serving:
Calories: 32, SmartPoints: 1

Ingredients
- 1 large onion, sliced thinly
- 1 stalk celery, sliced
- 1 cup carrot, sliced
- 2 garlic cloves, minced
- 1 cup tomatoes, diced
- 2 ½ cup cabbage, shredded
- 1 can non-fat beef broth
- 2 beef bouillon cubes
- ½ teaspoon dried basil
- 1 teaspoon Cajun spice
- 1 1/2 cups water
- ½ cup zucchini, sliced

Instructions

1. Press the Sauté button on your Instant Pot.
2. Sauté the onion, celery and carrots for five minutes or until vegetables are tender
3. Add in the garlic, tomatoes, cabbage, beef broth, bouillon cubes, basil, and Cajun spice.
4. Add water last.
5. Close the lid of the Instant Pot and set the venting knob to the sealing position.
6. Press the Soup button and press the "+" "- " button to set the time to 5 minutes.
7. Do quick pressure release.
8. Set the Instant Pot to sauté and add the zucchini. Cook for another 5 minutes.

Low Fat Taco Soup

Yields: 10
Cooking time: 15 minutes
Preparation time: 5 minutes

Nutritional Information per Serving:
Calories: 246, SmartPoints: 6

Ingredients
- 1 pound turkey breasts, ground
- 1 large onion, chopped
- 3 tablespoon prepared ranch dressing
- 1 tablespoon taco seasoning mix
- 1 can pinto beans, undrained
- 1 can whole kernel corn, undrained
- 1 can hot chili beans, undrained
- 1 can tomatoes
- Salt and pepper to taste

Instructions

1. Press the Sauté button on the Instant Pot.
2. Put the turkey meat and onions and cook until the turkey fat has rendered. Discard the excess fat.
3. Add the ranch dressing and taco seasoning mix. Mix until well combined.

4. Add the undrained pinto beans, corn, chili beans and stewed tomatoes.
5. Close the lid and make sure that the Instant Pot is sealed.
6. Press the stew button and adjust the timer by pressing the "+" "-" button. Adjust the time for 10 minutes.
7. Do natural pressure release.
8. Season with salt and pepper to taste.

Five Can Soup

Yields: 6
Cooking time: 15 minutes
Preparation time: 5 minutes

Nutritional Information per Serving:
Calories:210, SmartPoints:5

Ingredients

- 1 can corn, undrained
- 1 can diced tomatoes
- 1 can soup, any kind
- 1 can mixed vegetables
- 1 can black beans
- Salt and pepper to taste

Instructions

1. Mix all ingredients in the Instant Pot.
2. Close the lid.
3. Select the manual button and cook on high for 10 minutes.
4. Do natural pressure release for 5 minutes and adjust the seasoning with salt and pepper.

Instant Pot Tomato Spinach Soup

Yields: 8
Cooking time: 10 minutes
Preparation time: 5 minutes

Nutritional Information per Serving:
Calories: 43, SmartPoints: 2

Ingredients
- 1 cup baby spinach, washed
- 2 medium carrots, chopped
- 1 large onion, chopped
- 2 stalks of celery, chopped
- 1 clove of garlic, minced
- 1 can tomatoes
- 2 bay leaves
- 1 tablespoon dried basil
- 1 tablespoon dried oregano
- 2 cups low sodium vegetable broth
- 1 teaspoon red pepper flakes
- Salt and pepper to taste

Instructions

1. Place all the ingredients in the Instant Pot.
2. Close the lid and press the Soup button. Cook on the preset setting.

3. Do quick pressure release and remove the bay leaves.
4. Adjust the seasoning by putting in more salt and pepper if needed.

French Onion Soup

Yields: 6
Cooking time: 20 minutes
Preparation time: 5 minutes

Nutritional Information per Serving:
Calories:331, SmartPoints:10

Ingredients
- 1 tablespoon canola oil
- 6 large onions, sliced
- 1 tablespoon all-purpose flour
- 3 sprig fresh thyme leaves
- 1 cup low sodium beef broth
- 1 ½ cup chicken broth
- ½ cup goat cheese
- Salt and pepper to taste
- 6 slices of French bread

Instructions

1. Press the Sauté button on the Instant Pot.
2. Pour the oil and sauté the onion until soft.
3. Add in flour and cook until the flour has lightly browned.
4. Mix in the thyme and pepper. Add in the broth.

5. Close the lid and press the manual button. Cook on low pressure for 10 minutes.
6. Do natural pressure release for 10 minutes.
7. Season with salt and pepper to taste.
8. Press the sauté and the cheese.
9. Serve with bread slices.

Cheeseburger Stew

Yields: 8
Cooking time: 20 minutes
Preparation time: 5 minutes

Nutritional Information per Serving:
Calories:208, SmartPoints: 7

Ingredients
- Cooking spray to coat the bottom of the pot
- 1 clove garlic, minced
- 1 onion, chopped
- 1 stalk celery, chopped
- 1 pound lean ground beef
- 1 ½ cups canned chicken broth
- 1 cup low-fat evaporated milk
- 8-ounces low fat cheddar cheese, cubed
- 1 teaspoon paprika
- Salt and pepper to taste
- 2 tablespoon all-purpose flour + 2 tablespoon water
- 24 baked tortilla chips

Instructions

1. Press the Sauté button on your Instant Pot.
2. Coat the inner pot with cooking spray.

3. Sauté garlic, onion, and celery. Cook until the vegetables are tender.
4. Add the beef and brown for a few minutes. Pour in the broth.
5. Stir in the milk, cheese, and paprika. Season with salt and pepper to taste.
6. Close the lid and press the manual button. Cook on high for 10 minutes.
7. Do quick pressure release. Meanwhile, mix together flour and water to make a slurry.
8. Once the lid is open, press the sauté button and add the slurry mixture.
9. Cook and let the stew thicken.
10. Serve with tortilla chips.

Instant Pot Broccoli Cheese Soup

Yields: 10
Cooking time: 5 minutes
Preparation time: 3 minutes

Nutritional Information per Serving:
Calories:112, SmartPoints: 3

Ingredients
- 3 cups frozen broccoli
- 3 cans chicken broth
- 1 can tomatoes
- 1 cup reduced fat cheddar cheese

Instructions

1. Add all the ingredients in your Instant Pot except the cheese.
2. Close the lid and select the manual button. Cook on high for 5 minutes.
3. Do quick release to open the lid.
4. Press the sauté button and add the cheese.
5. Simmer until the cheese has melted.

Cheesy Potato Soup with Bacon

Yields: 12
Cooking time: 20 minutes
Preparation time: 5 minutes

Nutritional Information per Serving:
Calories:159, SmartPoints: 5

Ingredients
- 4 slices of bacon, chopped
- 1 onion, diced
- 2 cans fat-free chicken broth
- 1 cup potatoes, diced
- 1 cup low fat cheddar cheese
- ¼ cup sour cream
- Salt and pepper to taste
- 2 tablespoon flour + 1 tablespoon water

Instructions

1. Press the sauté button on the Instant Pot.
2. Add the bacon and cook until the bacon has rendered its fat. Drain the excess fat then set the bacon aside.
3. Sauté the onion and add the potatoes.
4. Pour in the chicken broth then close the lid.

5. Press the manual button and cook on high for 15 minutes.
6. Do quick pressure release to open the lid.
7. Add the low-fat cheddar cheese and sour cream.
8. Season with salt and pepper to taste.
9. Add the flour slurry and let the sauce thicken for 5 more minutes.
10. Top with crispy bacon.

Cauliflower and Broccoli Soup

Yields: 6
Cooking time: 5 minutes
Preparation time: 5 minutes

Nutritional Information per Serving:
Calories:53, SmartPoints: 2

Ingredients

- 1 ½ cup cauliflower, chopped
- 1 ½ cup broccoli, chopped
- 1 cup carrots, chopped
- 1 large onion, chopped
- 1 teaspoon dried oregano
- 1 teaspoon dried basil
- 1 chicken bouillon cube
- 3 cups water
- Salt and pepper to taste

Instructions

1. Place all ingredients in the Instant Pot.
2. Cover the lid and make sure that it is sealed.
3. Press the manual button and cook on high for 5 minutes.
4. Do natural pressure release to open the lid.

5. Place the soup in a blender and pulse until smooth.

Baked Potato Soup

Yields: 6
Cooking time: 20 minutes
Preparation time: 5 minutes

Nutritional Information per Serving:
Calories: 271, SmartPoints:8

Ingredients
- 6 slices turkey bacon, chopped
- 1 bulb garlic, minced
- 3-pounds potatoes, chopped
- 1 ½ tablespoon fresh thyme
- Salt and pepper to taste
- 4 cups low sodium chicken broth
- 6 tablespoon sour cream
- 6 tablespoon cheddar cheese, shredded
- 6 tablespoon scallions

Instructions

1. Press the Sauté button on the Instant Pot and add the bacon. Cook until the bacon has browned and the fat has rendered. Drain the excess fat. Set aside.
2. Add the garlic and sauté for a few minutes until slightly browned.

3. Add the potatoes and stir in the thyme. Season with salt and pepper to taste.
4. Pour in the chicken broth.
5. Close the lid and make sure that it is tightly sealed.
6. Press the manual button and cook on high for 15 minutes.
7. Do natural pressure release.
8. Ladle the soup onto bowls and top with sour cream, cheese, bacon and scallions.

Broccoli Potato Cheese Chowder

Yields: 6
Cooking time:
Preparation time:

Nutritional Information per Serving:
Calories:415, SmartPoints: 13

Ingredients
- ¾ cup celery, chopped
- ¼ cup onion, chopped
- ¼ cup parsley, chopped
- 2 cups potato, cubed
- ¾ cup carrots, chopped
- 1 cup broccoli, chopped
- 1 black pepper
- 1 ounce ham
- 1 cup water
- 2 bouillon cubes
- 2 tablespoon flour
- 1 cup milk
- ¼ cup low fat cheddar cheese

Instructions

1. Place the celery, onion, parsley, potatoes, carrots, broccoli, and pepper in the Instant Pot.

2. Stir in the ham
3. Pour in water and bouillon cubes.
4. Close the lid and press the manual button. Cook on high for 10 minutes.
5. Do quick pressure release to open the lid.
6. Press the Sauté button and whisk in the flour and milk. Stir to remove the lumps and until the sauce thickens.
7. Add the cheese last.

Egg Drop Soup with Chicken

Yields: 5
Cooking time: 15 minutes
Preparation time: 5 minutes

Nutritional Information per Serving:
Calories:119, SmartPoints: 3

Ingredients
- 4 cups chicken broth
- ½ teaspoon soy sauce
- ½ cup skinless chicken breast, chopped
- ¼ cup green onion, sliced
- ½ cup frozen green peas
- 1 egg lightly beaten.
- Salt and pepper to taste

Instructions
1. Place all ingredients in the Instant Pot except the egg.
2. Close the lid and press the manual button.
3. Cook on high for 10 minutes.
4. Do quick pressure release to open the lid.
5. Press the sauté button and let the soup get hot enough before adding the beaten egg. Let it sit for a minute for the egg to set.
6. Season with salt and pepper to taste.

Chicken Recipes

Parmesan Chicken with Mushroom and Wine Sauce

Yields: 4
Cooking time: 10 minutes
Preparation time: 5 minutes

Nutritional Information per Serving:
Calories:298, SmartPoints:8

Ingredients
- 2 tablespoon flour
- 2 tablespoon parmesan cheese, grated
- ½ teaspoon salt, divided
- ¼ teaspoon pepper
- 16 ounces of chicken breasts
- 1 tablespoon oil
- 2 cups onion, diced
- 2 garlic cloves, minced
- 2 cups mushroom, sliced
- ½ teaspoon dried basil
- 1 cup water
- 2 tablespoon dry wine

Instructions

1. Combine together the flour, parmesan cheese, and ¼ teaspoon each of salt and pepper.
2. Dredge the chicken and set aside.
3. Press the Sauté button on the Instant Pot and add 1 ½ teaspoon oil and sear the chicken for two minutes on both sides. Add the onions and garlic until wilted.
4. Stir in the mushrooms, basil, and the remaining salt. Cook until the mushrooms are tender.
5. Add water and wine.
6. Close the lid and press the manual button. Cook the chicken on high for five minutes.
7. Do natural pressure release.

Instant Pot Sweet and Sour Chicken

Yields: 4
Cooking time: 10 minutes
Preparation time: 5 minutes

Nutritional Information per Serving:
Calories:206, SmartPoints:7

Ingredients
- Cooking spray to coat the inner pot
- 1 pound boneless chicken breast
- ¼ teaspoon onion powder
- ¼ teaspoon garlic powder
- 5 ounce sweet and sour sauce
- 1 tablespoon brown sugar
- 8-ounces pineapple chunks
- 16 ounces of mixed frozen vegetables

Instructions

1. Coat the inner pot of your Instant Pot with cooking spray.
2. Press the Sauté button and add the chicken, onion powder, and garlic powder.
3. Add in the sweet and sour sauce, brown sugar, and pineapple chunks with juice.
4. Stir in the frozen vegetables.

5. Close the lid and press the manual button. Cook on high pressure for 7 minutes.
6. Do quick release to open the lid.

Steamed Jalapeno Chicken

Yields: 4
Cooking time: 10 minutes
Preparation time: 8 hours

Nutritional Information per Serving:
Calories:202, SmartPoints: 5

Ingredients
- ½ cup jalapeno jelly, melted
- ½ cup steak sauce
- 1 teaspoon garlic powder
- 2 tablespoon low-sodium Worcestershire sauce
- 4-ounces boneless chicken breasts, skin removed

Instructions

1. In a bowl, mix together the jalapeno jelly, steak sauce, garlic powder and Worcestershire sauce.
2. Marinate the chicken for at least 8 hours.
3. Remove the chicken from the bag and remove the marinade.
4. Place a steamer inside the Instant Pot and add the chicken pieces. Add 1 cup of water.
5. Close the lid and press the manual button. Cook on high for 10 minutes.
6. Do quick pressure release

Steamed Coconut Chicken with Pina Colada Dip

Yields: 4
Cooking time: 10 minutes
Preparation time: 1 hour and 30 minutes

Nutritional Information per Serving:
Calories:301, SmartPoints: 16

Ingredients
- 1 tablespoon lime juice
- 14 ounces can light coconut milk
- 1 tablespoon hot pepper sauce
- 1 pound boneless chicken, skin removed
- ¼ cup bread crumbs
- ½ cup sweetened flaked coconut
- ½ teaspoon salt
- ¼ teaspoon black pepper, ground
- 3-ounces crushed pineapple
- 3-ounces fat-free sour cream
- 4-ounces Pina colada non-alcoholic drink mixer

Instructions

1. Prepare the coconut chicken by mixing the lime juice, light coconut milk, and hot pepper sauce.
2. Add the chicken and marinate for 1 ½ hours.

3. In another bowl, combine the bread crumbs and coconut. Season with salt and pepper.
4. Dredge the chicken in the coconut flakes mixture.
5. Place the trivet or steam rack in the Instant Pot and add 1 ½ cup of water.
6. Close the lid and steam the chicken. Press the manual button and cook on high for 10 minutes.
7. Prepare the Pina colada dip by mixing the pineapple, sour cream and drink mixer.
8. Serve with the chicken.

Instant Pot Roast Chicken

Yields: 6
Cooking time: 20 minutes
Preparation time: 10 minutes

Nutritional Information per Serving:
Calories: 178, SmartPoints: 5

Ingredients
- 1 large roasting chicken
- 2 teaspoon extra-virgin olive oil
- 2 cloves of garlic, minced
- 2 teaspoon fresh thyme
- 1 teaspoon black pepper
- 1 teaspoon paprika
- 1 teaspoon sea salt
- 2 stalks celery, chopped
- 1 cup baby carrots
- 1 ½ cup water
- 2 medium potatoes, cubed

Instructions

1. Rub the chicken with olive oil, garlic, thyme, black pepper, paprika and salt.
2. Place the celery and baby carrots inside the cavity of the chicken.

3. Place the chicken in the Instant Pot and pour in the water. Add the baby potatoes around the chicken.
4. Close the lid and press the manual button. Cook on high for 20 minutes.
5. Do natural pressure release.
6. Take the chicken and potatoes out from the Instant Pot and press the sauté button.
7. Simmer the sauce until the sauce reduces and thickens.
8. Serve the chicken with the sauce.

Steamed Chicken Pot Pie

Yields: 4
Cooking time: 10 minutes
Preparation time: 5 minutes

Nutritional Information per Serving:
Calories:230, SmartPoints: 10

Ingredients
- ½ cup skim milk
- 2 eggs
- 1 cup baking mix (i.e. Bisquick)
- 2 cups cooked boneless chicken breast
- 2 cups frozen mixed vegetables
- 2 can low-sodium mushroom soup
- Salt and pepper to taste

Instructions

1. In a bowl, mix the milk, egg and baking mix. Set aside.
2. In another bowl, mix the chicken, frozen vegetables and cream of mushroom soup. Season with salt and pepper to taste.
3. Place chicken mixture in a ramekin and top with the batter.

4. Place a steam rack in the Instant Pot and add 1 cup water.
5. Place the ramekins inside the pressure cooker and close the lid.
6. Press the manual button and steam for 10 minutes.
7. Do quick pressure release to remove the lid.

Chicken Steak

Yields: 4
Cooking time: 10 minutes
Preparation time: 10 minutes

Nutritional Information per Serving:
Calories:224, SmartPoints: 11

Ingredients

- 4-pieces lean chicken breast, cut into steak
- ½ cup low-fat buttermilk
- 1 cup flour
- 1 teaspoon salt
- 1 teaspoon steak seasoning
- 2 tablespoon oil

Instructions

1. Dip the chicken steak in buttermilk.
2. In another bowl, combine the flour, salt, and steak seasoning.
3. Dredge the chicken steak in the flour mixture.
4. Press the Sauté button on the Instant Pot.
5. Place oil in the Instant Pot and add in the chicken pieces.
6. Cook for 5 minutes on each side.
7. Serve with ketchup or commercial gravy.

Steamed Lemon Chicken Breast

Yields: 4
Cooking time: 16 minutes
Preparation time: 5 minutes

Nutritional Information per Serving:
Calories:139, SmartPoints: 3

Ingredients

- 2 tablespoon lemon pepper seasoning
- 1 tablespoon all-purpose flour
- 4-pieces boneless chicken, skin removed
- 1 tablespoon unsalted butter
- ½ medium lemon, zest and juiced
- 1 cup low-sodium chicken broth

Instructions

1. In a shallow plate, mix together the lemon pepper seasoning and flour.
2. Dredge the chicken with the flour mixture.
3. Press the Sauté button on the Instant Pot and add unsalted butter. Add the chicken pieces and cook for 3 minutes on each side.
4. Pour over the lemon zest and juice. Add the broth.
5. Close the lid and press the manual button. Cook on high for 10 minutes.
6. Do natural release to remove the lid.

Sesame Chicken

Yields: 4
Cooking time: 13 minutes
Preparation time: 10 minutes

Nutritional Information per Serving:
Calories:216, SmartPoints: 4

Ingredients
- 2 tablespoon raw sesame seeds
- 1 tablespoon water
- 1 tablespoon low-sodium soy sauce
- 1 tablespoon maple syrup
- 1 teaspoon ginger root, grated
- ½ teaspoon five-spice powder
- 1 tablespoon dry sherry
- Salt and pepper to taste
- 1 pound boneless chicken breast, skin removed
- 1 cup water
- 2 tablespoon peanut oil

Instructions

1. Press the Sauté button on the Instant Pot.
2. Toast the sesame seeds for 3 minutes. Continue on stirring the sesame seeds to avoid over browning. Set aside.

3. In another pot, combine water, soy sauce, and maple syrup. Add the ginger, five-spice powder and sherry.
4. In another dish, mix the flour, salt and pepper.
5. Dredge the chicken with the flour mixture.
6. Press the Sauté button on your Instant Pot and add the chicken. Sauté until the sides have browned.
7. Add the soy sauce mixture. Pour in 1 cup water.
8. Close the lid and press the manual button. Cook on high for 10 minutes.
9. Do natural release to open the lid.
10. Press the sauté button and simmer until the sauce thickens.
11. Toss the sesame seeds to coat the chicken and add peanut oil.

Instant Pot Teriyaki Chicken

Yields: 6
Cooking time: 15 minutes
Preparation time: 5 minutes

Nutritional Information per Serving:
Calories:318, SmartPoints: 9

Ingredients

- 2 ½ pounds boneless chicken breast, skin removed
- ½ cup honey
- ½ cup soy sauce
- 1 tablespoon hot chili sauce
- 3 whole garlic cloves
- 1 cup water

Instructions

1. Place the chicken in the Instant Pot and add the honey, soy sauce, hot chili sauce and garlic cloves. Pour in water.
2. Close the lid and press the manual button. Cook on high for 10 minutes.
3. Do natural pressure release to open the lid.
4. Press the Sauté button and let the sauce simmer for 5 minutes until it thickens.

Instant Pot Curried Lemon Coconut Chicken

Yields: 6
Cooking time: 10 minutes
Preparation time: 5 minutes

Nutritional Information per Serving:
Calories:215, SmartPoints: 7

Ingredients
- ¼ cup lemon juice
- 1 can full-fat coconut milk
- 1 tablespoon curry powder
- 1 teaspoon turmeric
- ½ teaspoon lemon zest
- ½ teaspoon salt
- 4-pounds chicken breast, skin removed

Instructions
1. In a bowl, mix together the lemon juice, coconut milk, curry powder, turmeric, lemon zest and salt.
2. Place the chicken inside the Instant Pot and pour over the sauce mixture.
3. Close the lid.
4. Press the poultry button and cook on the preset setting.
5. Do natural release.

One Pot Chicken Cacciatore

Yields: 4
Cooking time: 18 minutes
Preparation time: 5 minutes

Nutritional Information per Serving:
Calories: 418, SmartPoints: 11

Ingredients

- 1 pound boneless chicken breast, skin removed
- ½ teaspoon salt
- ¼ teaspoon black pepper
- 1 teaspoon olive oil
- 1 medium onion, chopped
- 1 medium yellow pepper, chopped
- 1 medium green pepper, chopped
- 1 clove of garlic, chopped
- ½ cup broth
- 1 can tomatoes
- 1 tablespoon fresh parsley

Instructions

1. Season the chicken with salt and pepper.
2. Press the Sauté button on the Instant Pot and add the oil.

3. Add the chicken and brown the sides for 3 minutes.
4. Stir in the onions, pepper, and garlic and cook until the vegetables are soft.
5. Add the rest of the ingredients except the parsley.
6. Close the lid and press the manual button. Cook on high for 15 minutes.
7. Do quick pressure release to open the lid.
8. Garnish with parsley.

Beef Recipes

Instant Pot Caribbean Pineapple Filet Mignon

Yields: 1
Cooking time: 35 minutes
Preparation time: 5 minutes

Nutritional Information per Serving:
Calories:246, SmartPoints: 9

Ingredients
- 1 filet mignon
- ½ cup pineapple, chopped
- 1 piece bacon
- ¼ teaspoon jalapeno pepper
- 2 tablespoon red onions, chopped
- 4 tablespoon olive oil
- 2 cloves of garlic, minced
- 2 tablespoon coconut aminos or soy sauce
- 3 tablespoon honey
- ½ of a lime, juiced
- 1 tablespoon apple cider vinegar
- ¼ teaspoon ground ginger
- 1 teaspoon thyme
- ¼ teaspoon cinnamon

- 1/8 teaspoon ground cloves
- 1/8 teaspoon ground nutmeg
- Salt and pepper to taste

Instructions

1. Place all ingredients in the Instant Pot and mix well.
2. Close the lid and press the manual button. Cook on high for 35 minutes.
3. Do natural pressure release to open the lid.

Ground Beef and Cabbage Casserole

Yields: 8
Cooking time: 25 minutes
Preparation time: 10 minutes

Nutritional Information per Serving:
Calories: 249, SmartPoints: 8

Ingredients

- 1 pound lean ground beef
- ½ cup onion, chopped
- ½ cup uncooked brown rice
- 1 can tomato sauce
- 1 cube beef bouillon
- 1 tablespoon Worcestershire sauce
- 1 teaspoon sugar
- ½ teaspoon dried dill
- 1 cup water
- 4 cups cabbage, finely chopped
- 6-ounces Swiss cheese, grated

Instructions

1. Press the Sauté button on the Instant Pot.
2. Add the ground beef and onions and sauté until the beef has browned and rendered some fat. Remove excess fat.

3. Add the rice, tomato sauce, beef bouillon, Worcestershire sauce, sugar, and dill. Mix together until well combined. Pour in water.
4. Cover the lid and press the manual button. Cook on high for 15 minutes.
5. Do natural release for 10 minutes to open the lid.
6. Once the lid is open, add the cabbage and press the sauté button. Mix the rice and cabbages until the cabbages have wilted.
7. Top with cheese.

Instant Pot Meatloaf

Yields: 4
Cooking time: 25 minutes
Preparation time: 15 minutes

Nutritional Information per Serving:
Calories:240, SmartPoints: 7

Ingredients
- ¼ cup onion, chopped
- 1 pound lean ground beef
- 2 large egg whites
- ¼ cup seasoned Italian bread crumbs
- ½ cup barbecue sauce, divided

Instructions

1. In a mixing bowl, combine onion, meat, egg whites, and bread crumbs. Season with ¼ of the barbecue sauce.
2. Shape the mixture into a log and place them on parchment paper. Make sure that it will fit inside the Instant Pot.
3. Place a trivet or steam rack in the instant pot and add 1 ½ cups of water.
4. Set the meatloaf on top of the steam rack.

5. Close the lid and press the manual button. Cook on high for 25 minutes.
6. Do quick pressure release to remove the meatloaf.
7. Let it cool for one hour before pouring the remaining sauce on top.
8. You also have an option to broil it in the oven for 15 minutes to achieve browning.

Instant Pot Lasagna

Yields: 6
Cooking time: 20 minutes
Preparation time: 10 minutes

Nutritional Information per Serving:
Calories:360, SmartPoints: 11

Ingredients
- 1 pound lean ground beef
- 1 clove of garlic, minced
- 1 onion, chopped
- 1 can tomato sauce
- 1 can tomato, crushed
- 1 teaspoon salt
- $1/2$ teaspoon dried basil
- 1 teaspoon dried oregano
- $1/4$ teaspoon red pepper flakes
- $1^{1}/_{2}$ cup low-fat mozzarella cheese, grated
- 1 cup part-skim ricotta cheese
- 6 lasagna noodle
- ½ cup water
- $1/2$ cup parmesan cheese, grated

Instructions

1. Press the Sauté button on the Instant Pot and add the ground beef, garlic and onions. Stir constantly to avoid browning at the bottom and also to break up large pieces of the beef.
2. Add in the tomato sauce and crushed tomatoes. Season with salt, dried basil, oregano, and red pepper flakes. Set aside to assemble the lasagna.
3. Prepare the cheese sauce by mixing the 1 cup of mozzarella with ricotta.
4. Break the lasagna noodles and stir in the pot.
5. Place ¾ cup of the meat mixture at the bottom of the pot then drizzle with the cheese sauce. Add a layer of lasagna noodles. Do this alternately until all ingredients are placed inside the pot. Pour over water.
6. Close the lid and press the manual button. Cook on high for 15 minutes.
7. Do natural release to open the lid.
8. Sprinkle with parmesan cheese for garnish.

Beef Taco Rice

Yields: 4
Cooking time: 20 minutes
Preparation time: 5 minutes

Nutritional Information per Serving:
Calories:601, SmartPoints: 16

Ingredients
- 1 pound lean ground beef
- 1 onion, chopped
- 1 green bell pepper, chopped
- 1 cup long-grain white rice
- 1 packet taco seasoning mix
- ½ cup water
- 2 cups beef stock
- ¾ cup corn
- Salt and pepper to taste
- 1 ½ cup salsa
- 1 fresh cilantro, chopped

Instructions

1. Press the Sauté button on the Instant Pot.
2. Add the ground beef, onions, and bell pepper. Cook for 3 minutes

3. Stir in the rice and mix together. Season with taco seasoning.
4. Pour in water and the beef stock. Mix in the corn until well combined. Season with salt and pepper to taste.
5. Close the lid and press the manual button. Cook on high for 15 minutes.
6. Do natural pressure release to open the lid.
7. Top the taco rice with salsa and cilantro.

Herb-Crusted Beef

Yields: 12
Cooking time: 35 minutes
Preparation time: 5 minutes

Nutritional Information per Serving:
Calories:405, SmartPoints: 6

Ingredients
- 1 pound lean beef roast
- ½ teaspoon black pepper, ground
- 1 ½ teaspoon salt
- ¼ cup Dijon mustard
- 1 ½ teaspoon prepared horseradish
- 2 tablespoon low-calorie mayonnaise
- 2 cloves of garlic, minced
- 1 ½ cup water
- 1/3 cup fresh parsley, chopped
- 2 tablespoon thyme, chopped
- 2 tablespoon dill, chopped

Instructions
1. Mix all ingredients in the Instant Pot.
2. Close the lid and press the manual button. Cook on high for 35 minutes.
3. Do natural pressure release.
4. Check if the meat is done and tender.

Instant Pot Mexican Beef

Yields: 4
Cooking time: 25 minutes
Preparation time: 15 minutes

Nutritional Information per Serving:
Calories: 508, SmartPoints: 13

Ingredients
- 1 pound lean beef
- 1 cup onion, chopped
- 1 can diced tomatoes, drained
- 1 can black beans, drained
- 1 ½ cup frozen corn
- 1 teaspoon red pepper flakes
- 1 cup water
- 1 cup fat-free sour cream
- ½ cup low-fat cheddar cheese, grated

Instructions

1. Press the Sauté button on the Instant Pot and add the ground beef and onions. Stir until the big lumps are removed. Add in the tomatoes, black beans, corn, and red pepper flakes. Pour in water.
2. Close the lid and press the manual button. Cook on high for 15 minutes.

3. Do natural pressure release.
4. Once the lid is open, press the Sauté button and add in the sour cream. Simmer for another 10 minutes until the sauce has reduced.
5. Sprinkle with cheese on top.

Instant Pot Salisbury Steak

Yields: 4
Cooking time: 10 minutes
Preparation time: 5 minutes

Nutritional Information per Serving:
Calories:225, SmartPoints: 5

Ingredients
- 1 pound lean ground beef
- ¼ teaspoon garlic powder
- ½ teaspoon salt
- ¼ teaspoon black pepper
- 1 cup mushrooms, diced
- ¼ cup onion, minced
- 1 teaspoon dried thyme
- 2 tablespoon dry sherry
- ½ cup beef gravy
- 1 cup water
- 2 tablespoon flour + 1 tablespoon water

Instructions

1. In a mixing bowl, mix together beef and garlic. Season with salt and pepper.
2. Shape into thick patties.

3. Press the Sauté button of the Instant Pot and spray with cooking oil. Add the patties and cook for 4 minutes on each side.
4. Add the mushrooms, onions, thyme and white wine.
5. Close the lid and press the manual button. Cook on high for three minutes.
6. Do a quick release to open the lid.
7. Press the Sauté button and add the beef gravy. Let it simmer for five minutes.
8. Add the flour and water slurry and cook for another 3 minutes until the sauce thickens.

Beef Stroganoff

Yields: 4
Cooking time: 25 minutes
Preparation time: 10 minutes

Nutritional Information per Serving:
Calories:279, SmartPoints: 8

Ingredients

- 6-ounces sirloin steak, fat-trimmed and cut into strips
- 1 ½ cup mushrooms, sliced
- ½ cup onion, chopped
- 3 cloves of garlic, chopped
- 1 cup beef broth
- ¼ cup tomato sauce
- 3 tablespoon sherry wine
- ¾ tablespoon Worcestershire sauce
- ¼ teaspoon salt
- ¼ teaspoon pepper
- 1/3 cup sour cream
- 1 cup dry medium egg noodles
- 2 teaspoon fresh parsley, chopped

Instructions

1. Press the Sauté button and cook the steak for 3 minutes. Add the mushroom, onion, and garlic and cook for another two minutes.
2. Pour in the broth, tomato sauce, sherry wine, and Worcestershire sauce. Season with salt and pepper to taste.
3. Close the lid and press the manual button. Cook on high for 25 minutes.
4. Do quick pressure release.
5. Once the lid is open, press the sauté button and add the sour cream and noodles.
6. Cook for 7 to 10 more minutes until the noodles are done.
7. Garnish with parsley.

Barbacoa Beef

Yields: 9
Cooking time: 40 minutes
Preparation time:

Nutritional Information per Serving:
Calories:153, SmartPoints: 3

Ingredients
- ½ medium onion, chopped
- 5 cloves of garlic, minced
- 1 tablespoon ground cumin
- 1 lime, juiced
- 4 tablespoon chipotles in adobo sauce
- 1 tablespoon ground oregano
- ½ teaspoon ground cloves
- 1 cup water
- 3-pounds beef eye or round roast with fat trimmed
- 2 ½ teaspoon salt
- Black pepper to taste
- 1 teaspoon oil
- 3 bay leaves

Instructions

1. Place onion, garlic, cumin, lime juice, chipotles, oregano, and cloves in a blender. Add water and blend until smooth.
2. Season the beef with salt and pepper.
3. Press the Sauté button on the Instant Pot and heat the oil.
4. Add the beef and cook for 5 minutes until it turns brown on all sides.
5. Add the puree and bay leaves.
6. Close the lid and cook for 35 minutes.
7. Do quick pressure release.
8. Remove the beef and shred using a fork. Discard the bay leaves.
9. Return the shredded meat into the pot and adjust the seasoning.

Tomato Beef Macaroni Soup

Yields: 8
Cooking time: 25 minutes
Preparation time: 10 minutes

Nutritional Information per Serving:
Calories: 251, SmartPoints: 5

Ingredients
- 1 pound lean ground beef
- 1 ½ cups onion, chopped
- 2 cloves of garlic, chopped
- 1 can low-sodium beef broth
- 1 tablespoon Worcestershire sauce
- 1 can chopped tomatoes
- 1 jar pasta sauce
- 1 medium red bell pepper, chopped
- 1 cup frozen spinach
- 3 cups cooked elbow macaroni.

Instructions

1. Press the Sauté button on the Instant Pot.
2. Place the ground beef in the pot and cook until it has rendered some of its oil.
3. Add the onions and garlic. Sauté for another 3 minutes.

4. Add the beef broth and scrape the bottom to remove the crust or browning.
5. Add the rest of the ingredients except for the spinach and pasta.
6. Close the lid and cook on high for 20 minutes.
7. Do natural release.
8. Once the lid is open, press the Sauté button and add the spinach and pasta. Simmer for three minutes.

Tropical Beef with Peppers and Pineapple

Yields: 4
Cooking time: 20 minutes
Preparation time: 10 minutes

Nutritional Information per Serving:
Calories:405, SmartPoints: 9

Ingredients
- 1 tablespoon olive oil
- 1 large onion, chopped
- 2-pounds round steak, cut into chunks
- ½ teaspoon salt
- 1/8 teaspoon pepper
- 1 can pineapple chunks
- 2 large green peppers, chopped
- 1 can mild green chilies
- 1 can diced tomatoes
- 1 ½ tablespoon Greek seasoning
- 1 cup water
- 2 tablespoon cornstarch + 1 tablespoon water

Instructions

1. Press the Sauté button and heat the oil. Sauté the onion until tender. Keep on stirring to avoid the onions from burning.
2. Season the round steak with salt and pepper. Add to the pot and brown for another five minutes.
3. Add the pineapples, green pepper, chilis and diced tomatoes. Season with Greek seasoning. Add water.
4. Close the lid and press the stew button for 15 minutes.
5. Meanwhile, mix together the cornstarch and water in a bowl.
6. Do a quick release to open the lid. Add the cornstarch slurry and press the sauté button. Simmer until the sauce thickens.

Pork Recipes

Steamed Pork Tenderloin with Herbs

Yields: 8
Cooking time: 25 minutes
Preparation time: 35 minutes

Nutritional Information per Serving:
Calories:151, SmartPoints: 3

Ingredients

- 2 teaspoon dried oregano
- 2 teaspoon dried thyme
- 1 teaspoon onion powder
- 1 teaspoon garlic powder
- 1 teaspoon table salt
- 1 teaspoon black pepper
- 2 teaspoon olive oil
- 2-pounds lean pork tenderloin

Instructions

1. In a small mixing bowl, mix together oregano, thyme, onion powder, garlic powder, salt, and pepper.

2. Rub oil over the pork and sprinkle the herb mixture.
3. Let it rest for 30 minutes.
4. Place a steamer in the Instant Pot and place the marinated pork.
5. Add 1 cup of water to generate steam.
6. Close the lid. Press the manual button and cook on high for 25 minutes.
7. Do quick pressure release.

Southwestern Pork Chops

Yields: 4
Cooking time: 20 minutes
Preparation time: 10 minutes

Nutritional Information per Serving:
Calories: 184, SmartPoints:4

Ingredients
- 4-ounces lean pork loin chop, boneless and fat trimmed
- 1 vegetable oil
- 1/3 cup salsa
- 2 tablespoon lime juice
- 1 cup water
- ¼ cup fresh cilantro

Instructions
1. Flatten the pork chops with your hand.
2. Add oil to the Instant Pot set at the sauté setting. Place the pork chops and cook for one minute on each side.
3. Pour the salsa and lime juice over the pork chops.
4. Add in the water.
5. Close the lid and press the stew setting. Press the "+" "-" button and adjust the time to 15 minutes.
6. Do natural pressure release.
7. Sprinkle with cilantro on top.

BBQ Pork Tenderloin with Mop Sauce

Yields: 6
Cooking time: 30 minutes
Preparation time: 10 minutes

Nutritional Information per Serving:
Calories:199, SmartPoints: 5

Ingredients
- 1 tablespoon paprika
- 2 tablespoon brown sugar
- 1 tablespoon chili powder
- 1 ½ teaspoon ground cumin
- ¼ teaspoon cayenne pepper
- 1 teaspoon salt
- 1 pepper, ground to taste
- 1 ½ pound pork tenderloin
- 1/3 cup ketchup
- ¼ cup apple cider vinegar
- 2 tablespoon molasses
- 2 teaspoon Worcestershire sauce

Instructions

1. Prepare the spice rub by mixing together paprika, brown sugar, chili powder, cumin, cayenne pepper, salt, and black pepper.

2. Rub the spice mix on to the pork.
3. Add a trivet or steam rack on the Instant Pot. Pour 1 cup of water on the Instant Pot.
4. Close the lid and press the manual button. Cook on high for 30 minutes.
5. Do quick pressure release.
6. Make the mop sauce by mixing the remaining ingredients in a bowl.
7. Pour the mop sauce over the steamed pork.

Pork Chop Stew

Yields: 4
Cooking time: 30 minutes
Preparation time: 10 minutes

Nutritional Information per Serving:
Calories: 392, SmartPoints: 6

Ingredients
- 4 pork chops
- Salt and pepper to taste
- 2 cloves of garlic, minced
- ¼ cup soy sauce
- ¼ cup chicken broth
- ¼ teaspoon red pepper flakes
- 1 tablespoon tapioca

Instructions

1. Press the sauté button on the Instant Pot.
2. Season the pork chops with salt and pepper.
3. Place the pork chops in the pot and cook for 2 minutes on both sides. Set the pork aside.
4. Add the garlic to the pot and add the rest of the ingredients except the tapioca flour.
5. Place the pork back into the pot.

6. Close the lid and press the manual button. Cook on high for 20 minutes.
7. Do quick pressure release to open the lid.
8. Press the sauté button and add the tapioca flour.
9. Simmer until the sauce thickens.

Instant Pot Balsamic Pork Roast

Yields: 8
Cooking time: 30 minutes
Preparation time: 5 minutes

Nutritional Information per Serving:
Calories: 214, SmartPoints: 4

Ingredients

- 2-pounds pork shoulder roast, bones removed
- ½ teaspoon garlic powder
- ½ teaspoon red pepper flakes
- Salt to taste
- 1/3 cup chicken broth
- 1/3 cup balsamic vinegar
- 1 tablespoon Worcestershire sauce
- 1 tablespoon honey

Instructions

1. Season the pork with garlic powder, red pepper flakes, and salt.
2. Place the pork in the Instant Pot. Pour the broth, vinegar, and Worcestershire sauce. Stir in the honey.
3. Close the lid and press the stew button. Cook on high for 25 minutes.

4. Do quick pressure release.
5. Take the meat out from the Instant Pot and shred the meat with fork.
6. Place the meat back to the Instant Pot and press the sauté button. Simmer for 5 minutes.

Pork Carnitas

Yields: 4
Cooking time: 30 minutes
Preparation time: 5 minutes

Nutritional Information per Serving:
Calories: 432, SmartPoints:8

Ingredients

- 2 ½ pound lean pork tenderloin
- ¾ teaspoon salt
- ½ teaspoon salt
- 1 onion, diced
- 4 cloves of garlic, minced
- 1 teaspoon oregano
- 1 teaspoon cumin
- 2 tablespoon chipotle pepper with adobo sauce
- ¾ cup light beer
- 1 bay leaf

Instructions

1. Season the pork with salt and pepper.
2. Add the pork to the Instant Pot and place the remaining ingredients.
3. Close the lid and press the manual button. Cook on high for 25 minutes.

4. Do quick pressure release to open the lid.
5. Take the pork out and shred using a fork.
6. Place the shredded pork on a baking tray and toast for 5 minutes in a preheated oven. Bake at 500 °F
7. Press the sauté button and let the sauce simmer until it thickens. Pour the sauce over the toasted shredded pork.

Teriyaki Pork Tenderloin

Yields: 6
Cooking time: 25 minutes
Preparation time: 10 minutes

Nutritional Information per Serving:
Calories:332, SmartPoints: 7

Ingredients

- 2 tablespoon olive oil
- 2-pounds pork tenderloin, cut into strips
- 4 cloves of garlic, minced
- ½ large onion, chopped
- 3 red chili pepper, chopped
- ¼ teaspoon black pepper
- ½ cup teriyaki sauce
- 1 cup chicken broth
- ¼ cup brown sugar

Instructions

1. Press the sauté button on the Instant Pot.
2. Heat the oil and add the tenderloins. Stir constantly for 5 minutes or until they become brown.
3. Add in garlic, onion, red chili pepper and black pepper.

4. Add the remaining ingredients.
5. Close the lid and press the stew button. Adjust the cooking time to 20 minutes.
6. Do natural pressure release.
7. Serve with rice.

Pork with Salsa

Yields: 4
Cooking time: 40 minutes
Preparation time: 10 minutes

Nutritional Information per Serving:
Calories:265, SmartPoints: 10

Ingredients

- 3-pounds boneless pork shoulder blade roast, fat trimmed
- 6 cloves of garlic, crushed
- 3 tablespoon jerk seasoning
- ½ teaspoon coarse salt
- 1 lime, juice squeezed
- ½ cup fresh orange juice
- 1 avocado, diced
- 1 ½ tablespoon red onion, chopped
- 2 ripe mangoes, peeled and chopped
- 3 tablespoon lime juice
- 2 tablespoon fresh cilantro, chopped
- Salt and pepper to taste

Instructions

1. Cut slits into the pork meat and stuff holes with crushed garlic.

2. Place a steamer in the Instant Pot and add 2 cups water.
3. Place the meat at the center of the steamer.
4. In a mixing bowl, combine jerk seasoning, salt, lime juice, and orange juice.
5. Pour the sauce over the pork.
6. Close the lid and press the manual button. Cook on high for 35 minutes.
7. Meanwhile, prepare the salsa by combining the remaining ingredients in a bowl.
8. Go back to the pork and do natural pressure release to remove the lid once you hear the beeping sound.
9. Take the pork out and shred using fork.
10. Serve the pork with the salsa.

Pork Tenderloin Green Chili

Yields: 6
Cooking time:
Preparation time:

Nutritional Information per Serving:
Calories: 253, SmartPoints: 5

Ingredients
- 2 cups kale, chopped
- 2 15-ounce cannellini beans, drained
- 2 cups chicken broth
- 1 4 ounce diced green chilies, drained
- 1 cup salsa verde
- 1 cup chopped green bell pepper
- 2 cups onion, chopped
- 1 tablespoon chili powder
- 1 tablespoon garlic, minced
- 1 teaspoon ground cumin
- 1 dried bay leaf
- ½ teaspoon dried oregano
- 12-ounces pork tenderloin, boneless and fat trimmed
- ½ cup cilantro, chopped

Instructions

1. In a blender, mix together kale, half of the cannellini beans and broth. Blend until smooth.
2. Transfer this mixture into the slow cooker and add the rest of the ingredients except the cilantro.
3. Close the lid and press the manual button. Cook on high for 25 minutes.
4. Do quick pressure release to open the lid.
5. Remove the bay leaf and transfer the pork in another bowl. Shred with fork.
6. Garnish with cilantro.

Apple Barbecue Ribs

Yields: 6
Cooking time: 35 minutes
Preparation time: 10 minutes

Nutritional Information per Serving:
Calories: 489, SmartPoints: 10

Ingredients
- 4 cups apple juice
- ½ cup apple cider vinegar
- 1 tablespoon salt
- 3-pounds rack of ribs
- ½ tablespoon garlic powder
- ½ tablespoon black pepper
- 1 cup Southern apple cider barbecue sauce
- ½ cup water

Instructions
1. Place all ingredients in the pot.
2. Make sure that the pork is coated with the sauce.
3. Close the lid and press the manual button. Adjust the cooking time by pressing the "+" "-" button to 25 minutes.
4. Do quick release. Remove the ribs from the pot and set it on a baking pan. Cover the baking pan with aluminum foil and place the ribs in the oven. Cook for 10 minutes at 400 °F.

Honey Balsamic Pork Roast

Yields: 8
Cooking time: 35 minutes
Preparation time: 5 minutes

Nutritional Information per Serving:
Calories: 256, SmartPoints: 5

Ingredients
- 2-pound pork roast, bones and fat removed
- ½ teaspoon garlic powder
- Salt and pepper to taste
- 1/3 cup balsamic vinegar
- 1/3 cup vegetable broth
- ¼ cup liquid aminos
- 1 tablespoon raw honey
- 1 ½ cup water

Instructions

1. Place the pork roast in the Instant Pot and sprinkle with garlic powder, salt, and pepper. Rub the spices on the pork.
2. Add the rest of the ingredients.
3. Close the lid and select the manual button. Cook on high for 35 minutes.
4. Do quick pressure release.

Apple Bacon BBQ Pulled Pork

Yields: 10
Cooking time: 40 minutes
Preparation time: 10 minutes

Nutritional Information per Serving:
Calories:195, SmartPoints: 5

Ingredients

- 4 slices of bacon, chopped
- 1 ½ cup onion, chopped
- 1 medium apple, chopped
- 1 ½ cup ketchup
- 3 tablespoon brown sugar
- 1/3 cup Worcestershire sauce
- 3 tablespoon apple cider vinegar
- 2 teaspoon salt
- 2-pounds pork tenderloin

Instructions

1. Press the sauté button on the Instant Pot and drop the chopped bacons. Cook until the bacon has rendered its fat. Set aside.
2. Sauté the onions and apples for a minute. Add the ketchup, brown sugar, Worcestershire sauce, and apple cider vinegar. Season with salt.

3. Add the pork tenderloin.
4. Close the lid and press the manual button. Cook on high for 35 minutes.
5. Do natural pressure release.
6. Remove the pork from the pot and shred using a fork.
7. Garnish with crispy bacon.

Dessert Recipes

Mini Flourless Peanut Butter Chocolate Cakes

Yields: 4
Cooking time: 15 minutes
Preparation time: 10 minutes

Nutritional Information per Serving:
Calories:105, SmartPoints: 3

Ingredients
- 1 can black beans, drained and rinsed
- ½ cup cocoa powder, unsweetened
- ½ cup egg whites
- 1/3 cup canned pumpkin
- 1/3 cup unsweetened applesauce
- ¼ cup brown sugar
- 1 teaspoon vanilla extract
- 1 ½ teaspoon baking powder
- ¼ teaspoon salt
- 3 tablespoon peanut butter baking chips

Instructions

1. Place all the ingredients except the peanut butter chips inside a food processor. Process until smooth.
2. Add the peanut butter chips and fold until evenly distributed within the batter.
3. Place the batter in a ramekin sprayed with cooking oil.
4. Place a steam rack in the Instant Pot and add 1 ½ cup water.
5. Place the ramekins with the batter onto the steamer rack.
6. Close the lid and press the manual button. Cook on high for 10 minutes.
7. Do natural pressure release.
8. Insert a toothpick in the middle of the cakes and check if it comes out clean.
9. Serve chilled.

Instant Pot Berry Cobbler

Yields: 4
Cooking time: 10 minutes
Preparation time: 10 minutes

Nutritional Information per Serving:
Calories: 199, SmartPoints: 6

Ingredients
- 30 ounces frozen mixed berries
- ½ cup granulated white sugar, divided
- 2 ½ cup commercial baking mix
- ½ cup light vanilla soy milk
- 3 tablespoon whipped butter
- 2 teaspoon cinnamon

Instructions

1. Prepare the filling by mixing berries with ¼ cup white sugar and ½ cup commercial baking mix.
2. In another bowl, prepare the topping by combining 2 cups commercial baking mix, soy milk, ¼ cup white sugar, butter and cinnamon.
3. Place the filling in ramekins. Add the topping mixture.

4. Place a trivet or steam rack at the bottom of the Instant Pot and pour 1 cup water.
5. Place the ramekins on the rack.
6. Close the lid and press the manual button. Cook on high for 10 minutes.
7. Do natural pressure release for 10 minutes.

Scalloped Peaches

Yields: 8
Cooking time: 15 minutes
Preparation time: 10 minutes

Nutritional Information per Serving:
Calories:104, SmartPoints: 2

Ingredients

- 8 cups peaches, thinly sliced
- ¼ cup brown sugar
- 1 teaspoon cinnamon
- 1/8 teaspoon salt
- ¼ cup butter

Instructions

1. Place the peaches in a mixing bowl and add brown sugar, cinnamon and salt. Toss to combine everything. Add butter and mix again.
2. Place the peaches inside ramekins.
3. Place a steamer rack in the Instant Pot.
4. Arrange the ramekins on the steamer rack.
5. Close the lid and press the manual button. Cook on high for 15 minutes.
6. Do natural pressure release.

Custard Cream Cheesecake

Yields: 6
Cooking time: 25 minutes
Preparation time: 15 minutes

Nutritional Information per Serving:
Calories: 344, SmartPoints: 16

Ingredients
- 1 ½ cup custard cream biscuits
- ¼ cup melted butter
- 2 cup full fat cream cheese
- ½ cup caster sugar
- 2 large eggs
- 1 teaspoon vanilla
- 2 drops of almond extract
- ¾ cup double cream

Instructions

1. Place the custard cream biscuits and butter in the food processor and pulse until a fine crumb is formed. This will be the dough
2. Press the dough in ramekins or small spring form pans.
3. Clean the food processor and pour in the cream cheese, caster sugar, eggs, vanilla extract, almond

extract, and double cream. Process until well combined.
4. Pour the mixture to the ramekins or cake pan. Place a kitchen towel on top of the ramekin to absorb the excess liquid from forming on the cheesecake
5. Pour 1 ½ cup of water to the Instant Pot and place a trivet. Place the ramekins or cake pan on the trivet.
6. Close the lid and select the manual button. Cook on high for 25 minutes.
7. Do natural pressure release then remove the lid. Remove the kitchen towel.
8. Refrigerate.

Instant Pot Applesauce

Yields: 8
Cooking time: 8 minutes
Preparation time: 5 minutes

Nutritional Information per Serving:
Calories: 96, SmartPoints: 5

Ingredients
- 8 medium apples, peeled and cored
- 1 cup water
- 2 teaspoon cinnamon, ground

Instructions

1. Place the apples in the Instant Pot. Pour in the water.
2. Close the lid and press the manual button. Cook on high for 8 minutes.
3. Do natural pressure release and open the lid.
4. Remove the excess water.
5. Place the apples in a blender and process until smooth.
6. Add the rest of the ingredients.
7. Serve chilled

Thai Coconut Rice

Yields: 4
Cooking time: 20 minutes
Preparation time: 10 minutes

Nutritional Information per Serving:
Calories: 102, SmartPoints: 4

Ingredients
- 1 cup Thai sweet rice
- 1 ½ cups water
- 1 can full fat coconut milk
- A pinch of salt
- 4 tablespoon pure sugar
- ½ teaspoon cornstarch + 2 tablespoon water
- 1 large mango, sliced
- Sesame seeds for garnish

Instructions

1. Place rice and water in the Instant Pot.
2. Close the lid and press the manual button. Cook on high for 5 minutes.
3. Turn off the Instant Pot and do natural pressure release for 10 minutes.

4. While the rice is cooking, place the coconut milk, salt, and sugar in a saucepan. Heat over medium heat for 10 minutes while stirring constantly.
5. Once the Instant Pot lid can be open, add the coconut milk mixture. Stir well. Place a clean kitchen towel over the opening of the lid and let it rest for 10 minutes.
6. Meanwhile, mix cornstarch with water and add to the rice. Press the sauté button and mix until the rice becomes creamy and thick.
7. Serve with mango slices and sesame seeds.

Toffee Pudding

Yields: 12
Cooking time: 20 minutes
Preparation time: 15 minutes

Nutritional Information per Serving:
Calories:305, SmartPoints: 16

Ingredients
- ¼ cup blackstrap molasses
- ¾ cup boiling water
- 1 ¼ cup dates, chopped
- 1 ¼ cup all-purpose flour
- ¼ teaspoon salt
- 1 teaspoon baking powder
- 1/3 cup unsalted butter + ¼ cup unsalted butter
- 1 ¾ cup brown sugar
- 1 egg
- 2 teaspoon vanilla extract
- 1/3 cup whipping cream

Instructions

1. Brush butter on ramekins and set aside.
2. In a bowl, mix together molasses, boiling water and dates. Mix in the flour, salt and baking soda. Place in a blender and pulse until fine.

3. In a separate bowl, cream the 1/3 cup butter and ¾ cup brown sugar using a hand mixer Do this until the butter becomes fluffy. Add the eggs and 1 teaspoon vanilla. Pour in the date mixture.
4. Divide the batter and distribute to the ramekins.
5. Cover the ramekins with foil and make sure that it is sealed well.
6. Place a steamer rack in the pressure cooker. Pour 2 cups of water.
7. Close the lid and press the manual button. Cook on high for 20 minutes.
8. Meanwhile, make the caramel sauce by mixing together the remaining vanilla, butter, and brown sugar. Add the whipping cream. Bring to a boil in a saucepan heated over medium low flame. Set aside.
9. Once the pudding is done, do quick natural release.
10. Remove the ramekins and pour the caramel sauce.

Apple Crisps

Yields: 4
Cooking time: 8 minutes
Preparation time: 5 minutes

Nutritional Information per Serving:
Calories:362, SmartPoints: 18

Ingredients
- 5 medium apples, peeled and chopped
- ½ teaspoon nutmeg
- 2 teaspoon cinnamon
- 1 tablespoon maple syrup
- ½ cup water
- 4 tablespoon butter
- ¾ cup old fashioned rolled oats
- ¼ cup brown sugar
- ¼ cup flour
- ½ teaspoon salt

Instructions

1. Place the apples in the Instant Pot and sprinkle with nutmeg and cinnamon. Pour in maple syrup and water.

2. In a small bowl, melt the butter in the microwave oven. Add to the melted butter oats, brown sugar, flour and salt.
3. Drop a spoonful of mixture on the apples.
4. Close the lid on the Instant Pot. Press the manual setting and cook on high for 8 minutes.
5. Use natural pressure release.
6. Serve warm and topped with vanilla ice cream.

Chocolate Berry Cheesecake

Yields: 16
Cooking time: 10 minutes
Preparation time: 25 minutes

Nutritional Information per Serving:
Calories:216, SmartPoints: 11

Ingredients
- 4 tablespoon butter, melted
- 1 ½ cup chocolate cookie, crumbed
- 3 packages low-fat cream cheese
- 2 tablespoon cornstarch
- 1 cup sugar
- 3 large eggs
- ½ cup plain Greek yogurt
- 1 tablespoon vanilla extract
- 4-ounce milk chocolate
- 4-ounce white chocolate
- 4-ounce bittersweet chocolate
- 1 cup sugared cranberries

Instructions

1. Brush ramekins or a spring form pan with oil. Set aside.

2. Make the crust by combining butter with cookie crumbs. Press the dough at the bottom of the pan. Place in the freezer to set.
3. Beat the cream cheese with a mixer on low speed until smooth. Add cornstarch and sugar and continue mixing until well combined. Mix in eggs one at a time while continuing to beat. Scrape the sides of the bowl as needed. Add the yogurt and vanilla and mix until well combined.
4. Divide the batter in three bowls. Set aside
5. Melt the milk chocolate in the microwave oven for 30 seconds twice until completely melted. Whisk the chocolate into one of the bowl of the cheesecake batter. Do the same thing with the white and bittersweet chocolates.
6. Take the spring form pan out from the fridge. Pour the dark chocolate batter as the first layer, followed by the white chocolate and milk chocolate. Put aluminum foil on top of the spring form pan.
7. Pour water on the Instant Pot and place the steamer rack. Place the spring form pan and close the lid.
8. Cook on high for 10 minutes.
9. Do natural pressure release to open the lid.
10. Take the cheesecake out and refrigerate for 1 hour.

11. Serve with sugared cranberries.

Molten Chocolate Mini Lava Cake

Yields: 3
Cooking time: 6 minutes
Preparation time: 10 minutes

Nutritional Information per Serving:
Calories:215, SmartPoints: 8

Ingredients

- 1 egg
- 4 tablespoon sugar
- 2 tablespoon olive oil
- 4 tablespoon milk
- 4 tablespoon all-purpose flour
- 1 tablespoon cacao powder
- ½ teaspoon baking powder
- Pinch of salt
- Powdered sugar for dusting

Instructions

1. Grease the ramekins with butter or oil. Set aside
2. Pour 1 cup of water in the Instant Pot and place the steamer rack.
3. In a medium bowl, mix all the ingredients except the powdered sugar. Blend until well combined.
4. Pour in the ramekins.

5. Place the ramekins in the Instant Pot and close the lid.
6. Press the manual button and cook on high for 6 minutes.
7. Once the Instant Pot beeps, remove the ramekin and sprinkle powdered sugar.

Pumpkin Banana Chocolate Chip Bundt Cake

Yields: 12
Cooking time: 35 minutes
Preparation time: 15 minutes

Nutritional Information per Serving:
Calories:120, SmartPoints: 4

Ingredients

- ¾ cup whole wheat flour
- ¾ cup all-purpose flour
- 1 teaspoon baking soda
- ½ teaspoon salt
- ½ teaspoon baking powder
- ¾ teaspoon pumpkin pie spice
- 1 medium banana, mashed
- ¾ cup sugar
- ½ cup Greek yogurt
- 2 tablespoon canola oil
- 1 egg
- ½ can pureed pumpkin
- ½ teaspoon vanilla extract
- 2/3 cup semi-sweet chocolate chips

Instructions

1. In a mixing bowl, mix together the two types of flour, baking soda, salt, baking powder, and pumpkin pie spice.
2. Using an electric mixer, combine the banana, sugar, yogurt, oil, egg, pureed pumpkin, and vanilla in a separate bowl.
3. Mix the dry ingredients and wet ingredients. Fold until well combined. Stir in the chocolate chips.
4. Transfer the batter in a greased Bundt pan.
5. Cover the pan with foil and make sure that it is sealed.
6. Add 1 ½ cups of water into the Instant Pot and place the steamer rack.
7. Place the Bundt pan on top of the rack.
8. Close the lid and press the manual button. Cook on high for 35 minutes.

Do natural pressure release.

Serve chilled.

Apple Bread with Salted Caramel Icing

Yields: 12
Cooking time: 35 minutes
Preparation time: 10 minutes

Nutritional Information per Serving:
Calories:314, SmartPoints:15

Ingredients
- 2 eggs
- 2 sticks butter
- 3 cup sugar
- 1 tablespoon apple pie spice
- 3 cups apples, peeled and cubed
- 2 cups flour
- 1 tablespoon baking powder
- 1 tablespoon vanilla
- 1 cup heavy cream
- 2 cups powdered sugar

Instructions

1. In a mixing bowl, combine the eggs, 1 stick butter, 1 cup sugar, and apple pie spice. Mix until creamy and smooth. Add in the apples and mix well.
2. In another bowl, mix together flour and baking powder. Add this mixture to the apple mixture.

Stir and pour the batter into a greased spring form pan.
3. Place a steamer rack in the Instant Pot and pour 1 ½ cup water. Place the pan on the trivet.
4. Close the lid and press the manual button. Cook on high for 35 minutes.
5. Do a natural pressure release.
6. Meanwhile, make the icing by mixing 1 stick butter, 2 cups sugar, heavy cream and powdered sugar. Heat over medium low flame.
7. Pour the icing on top of the apple bread.

Made in the USA
Lexington, KY
24 January 2018